A Better Normal for Chemotherapy

Your Guide to Rediscovering Intimacy After Cancer

Tess Devèze

CONTENTS

WHY I WROTE THIS BOOK

Hello! It's so wonderful to meet you. I'm Tess.

I thought before we get into the more 'intimate' details, I'd introduce myself and let you know what this book is about.

I was diagnosed with stage-three breast cancer in 2018, at the age of 36. At the time of my diagnosis, I'd been working in the sexuality sector for years. Over the years since my cancer diagnosis and endless treatments, only twice did a healthcare professional voluntarily bring up the topic of sexuality and only one booklet was recommended to me (which I had to go and find myself). The lack of information and support on this topic, both during and after treatments, was painfully noticeable.

Why aren't more resources available? Why are we so afraid to talk about this essential aspect of our lives?

First and foremost, I'm an occupational therapist (OT). What's an OT, I hear you ask? We are functional therapists and use specific approaches to promote independence and participation in 'occupations' which are any kind of meaningful life activity that occupies us. OT's help you do the day-to-day activities that you need and want to do, as best you can. This may include self-care tasks (shower, dressing, toileting), work related (vocational) tasks, social or community activities...and may also include sex!

My clinical experience is mostly in sexuality - during and after cancer treatments, brain-injury, neurological conditions, and those living with disability. Before moving solely to sexuality for people with cancer, disability and chronic illness, most of my work was in private and public hospitals across Australia, working in neurological rehabilitation. I love neuroscience, and most of my work is based on neurological concepts.

Other than having cancer and being a sexuality OT, I also work with sexuality and self-development pioneers 'Curious Creatures', based in Melbourne Australia. I've facilitated hundreds of workshops online and face to face for nearing a decade, teaching consent, better intimacy and communication skills. I've seen thousands of people's lives change through a deeper understanding of sexual intimacy.

Lastly, I've also studied somatic sexological bodywork at the Institute of Somatic Sexology. This training has given me a deeper understanding of how libido, pleasure, arousal and orgasmicity (cool word huh?) work on a physiological, neurological, and psychological level. These learnings form an essential part of this book.

Even with all my training, I've struggled. If you're struggling too, you're not alone (even if it doesn't get spoken about).

But it's not just about me. The contents of this book are also guided by you. I have a Facebook group 'Intimacy and Cancer' with thousands of people - all cancers, all genders - from over 49 countries, who share and support each other on this topic. My one-on-one clients have also been a huge source of learning, generously sharing their experiences.

It's been almost two years since releasing 'A Better Normal; Your Guide to Rediscovering Intimacy After Cancer', and the positive feedback I have personally been receiving from readers has been at times overwhelming. I am humbled, amazed and inspired by the impact and influence this book has had for those out there suffering.

But cancer treatments are *haaaaaard*, and so is reading! I wanted to know how I could reach more people, change more lives for the better through the contents in this book. In answer to that question, I've created the 'A Better Normal' mini-book *series*. It's a number of bite-sized treatment or side-effect specific mini-books, to help cancer patients and their loved ones maintain and grow connection, intimacy and sexuality. Each mini-book is created from the information in 'A Better Normal; Your Guide to Rediscovering Intimacy After Cancer', but broken down into simple, easy-to-read guides relative to your very specific needs, because often during and after treatments committing to a 300-page book feels overwhelming or is simply not possible.

Books in the 'A Better Normal' mini-book series are:

- 'A Better Normal for **Libido**; Your Guide to Rediscovering Intimacy After Cancer'
- 'A Better Normal for **Vaginal Dryness & Pain**; Your Guide to Rediscovering Intimacy After Cancer'
- 'A Better Normal for **Body Confidence**; Your Guide to Rediscovering Intimacy After Cancer'
- 'A Better Normal for **Chemotherapy**; Your Guide to Rediscovering Intimacy After Cancer'
- 'A Better Normal for **Hormone Therapy**; Your Guide to Rediscovering Intimacy After Cancer'
- 'A Better Normal for **Fatigue**; Your Guide to Rediscovering Intimacy After Cancer'

- 'A Better Normal for **Changes In Erection**; Your Guide to Rediscovering Intimacy After Cancer'
- 'A Better Normal for **Radiotherapy**; Your Guide to Rediscovering Intimacy After Cancer'
- 'A Better Normal for **Pain**; Your Guide to Rediscovering Intimacy After Cancer'

Or if you're after all of the above information (and more) in one place, the all-in-one book 'A Better Normal; Your Guide to Rediscovering Intimacy After Cancer' has everything you need.

If you end up with several mini-books in the series, that's pretty normal, as we don't have only one side-effect (geez, wouldn't that be nice!), and we can have the same side-effect from more than one treatment (like fatigue, or changes in libido). Cancer treatments impact us differently, which is why some books in this series are side-effect specific, and others treatment specific. So you can pick and choose what is most relevant for you and where you're at. You'll also notice that some mini-books have repeated information in them. That's because some information is essential and helpful, regardless of what your side-effect or treatment is (like the communication tips, or ways to gently reconnect with yourself or a partner).

The most important thing you can learn from this book is that you're not alone and you're not broken. There's nothing wrong with you if you're struggling. It's normal to find this situation tough. This isn't one-size-fits-all advice. All bodies are unique, every relationship is different, and everyone experiences relationships, connection, pleasure and desire in their own way. You're the expert on you! Just as cancer is different for everyone, so are the connections we have with ourselves and those around us.

Lastly, this book is for all human beings, regardless of gender, lifestyle, orientation, ability, ethnicity, age, or relationship dynamic. Although every person with cancer is unique, we have one thing in common: no matter who we are or what we are going through, we're all worthy of love and connection.

Now, let's get started on making your 'new normal', a 'better normal'.

1.   KEY TERMS EXPLAINED

Sexuality vs sex

The word 'sexuality' is an umbrella term which yes includes the functional activity of sex, but also includes relationships, connections, affection, dating, pleasure and our overall well-being. Sexuality can be greatly affected due to cancer, but it doesn't necessarily have to stop altogether. As a sexuality educator and clinician, I know how important sexuality, connection and intimacy is to our quality of life, our resilience and coping. What could be more important!

'Sex' in this book refers to the act, or the activity you engage in with yourself and/others, and is one of the most diverse and most adaptable functional activities I can think of. Yet today, it's still one of the most under-addressed topics in clinical settings. This is something I aim to change.

I also want us all to be on the same page in how we see 'sex' itself which is more than just orgasms and genital play, it's so much more. During cancer treatments and other life-altering events, you might need to temporarily let go of traditional forms of touch/sex. We can become excited, aroused, release pleasure hormones in our body from so many different ways. There are erogenous zones all over our bodies such as our inner thighs, breasts, nipples, under the armpits, the neck, earlobes, feet and many more depending on your body. Orgasms, engorgement, ejaculation, becoming 'hard' or 'wet', these don't need to be your goal, but can also be experienced in more than one way. Pleasure, enjoyment, arousal, excitation and connection, that is where the fun can also be. Pleasure is pleasurable and our whole body can be pleasured!

Desire vs arousal

Desire (the wanting) I use interchangeably with libido. Desire/libido are the experience of *wanting* sex and pleasure. Desire has many words that can be used, such as lust, sex-drive, and essentially all refer to that *want* we have.

Arousal is the way our body responds when it's in pleasure, the changes in our body that show us we are in fact, enjoying and excited. Things like increased sensitivity, maybe we become wet, maybe we become hard, our heart rate increases, we breathe heavier and more.

Simply put, libido = wanting, and arousal = enjoying.

Treatments can affect our arousal as well as our libido, which I dive into in this book, but knowing the difference between these can be very helpful.

The magical word, intimacy

Disconnection from yourself and others is a common side-effect of cancer treatments for so many. You're not alone in this and here I introduce you to the magical word 'intimacy'. Imagine that you having sex or being intimate again with yourself, a date or a partner/s, is the goal or the prize. That prize is on the other side of a river, and to get to it, you need to build a bridge. How can you do that? Through intimacy, through touch and the other magical word *affection*.

I've heard many times from clients and people in my support group "we don't even touch each other anymore". Not only has sex gone, but so has the *intimacy*, and are we really going to want sex without that connection?

Intimacy and affection are small giants. Tiny little things that can mean the world, and build that bridge of connection. Things like hand-holding, a good-night kiss, a good morning hug, your arm around your partner in the kitchen, cuddling on the couch, touch for the sake of touch (not as a way to 'get somewhere'), massage swaps, maybe a cheeky butt-squeeze and grin, and the big one, WORDS OF LOVE.

When you want some touch or love? Here's a few ways to ask, without that pressure of it needing to lead to sex:

How to say it out loud.

- "Hey, I'd like to be closer to you, how about a cuddle?"
- "Can we snuggle together on the couch while watching this film?"
- "You up for some hand-holding while we walk to the shop?"
- "I'm loving you right now, thought I'd share."
- "You up for some underwear-on cuddling while we fall asleep? I miss connecting with you."
- "I'd love some touch/to touch your body, would you like a massage?"
- "I'm not wanting this to lead to sex, but some kisses and cuddles would be lovely if you're feeling like some connection?"
- "I'm checking you out right now, just wanted to share."

- "I'm running a bath to relax and wind-down from the day, would you like to join me for some down-time?"

Small giant steps towards that prize.

2. CONNECTION

When people hear the word 'connection', some assume it means something to do with sex. Well, that is not necessarily always the case as there are so many different types of meaningful connection in our lives, which I'll discuss here.

Connection could be the sharing of intimacy through affection with another, or with yourself. It can make you warm, bring you closer to someone, provide feelings of value and being loved. A hug from a friend, a hand-hold from a family member, even a simple smile from a stranger. Connection, belonging, it all can have a positive impact on us.

Why connecting is essential

I want to share a 'light bulb' moment I had during chemotherapy, one that helped me change a lot about the way I connected to those around me.

I was 4 months into chemotherapy and had just switched to having chemo weekly. It was a sweltering 38-degree Australian summer night and I walked out of a poetry reading with a friend, to go home. While walking, he hooked his arm through mine, as a sign of affection and connection. When his arm linked through mine, I noticed that I jumped at the touch. Noticing my reaction and how much I had been startled at the contact, it dawned on me. How long had it been since I had been touched in a way that was not medical, hurried and detached? Three weeks? Maybe four? I was so used to the non-intimate hands of nurses, oncologists, surgeons etc. who were not aggressive, but let's say, purposefully unaffectionate in their touch. It was a shock to receive this wonderful soft, intimate connection of an arm slipping through mine. I realised I had become an object of analysis and procedure, and was no longer one of affection. It was shocking to me and it also saddened me.

That was the moment I realised I was losing connection, that was the moment I saw I was becoming detached and I needed to be more vocal. The people around me were being respectful and careful not to touch me, due to how unwell I was. I loved everyone's respectful approach and care towards me as I was very, very sick. I'm grateful for their care, but I realised they also needed guidance from me, to know what was okay and when.

Realising the only touch I had been receiving was

medical, which I would switch off to and detach myself from, was one of those 'ahaaa' moments. I had realised how disconnected I'd become to my body and that I needed to make the first move and communicate. So, I beg you, educate those around you. Tell your friends they can hold your hand, your family members can put their arm around you, a partner or lover can snuggle with you on the couch. Be their guide for your connection. There are some examples on how to do that further on in this book.

Our desires for physical intimacy change when we are stressed and unwell, that is a part of being human. However, it's important to mention here that chemotherapy, other treatments and the endless medications we take, can also affect our mind. 'Cancer-brain' also known as 'brain-fog' is actual cognitive dysfunction. It was and is, one of the most challenging side effects for me. Being unable to think, remember, concentrate, getting lost in my apartment building, losing my keys, forgetting the names of loved ones, it was and is scary. So, how do we give an invisible symptom, visibility? We speak of it, we give it voice, we give others' knowledge and understanding. It was difficult, but was helpful for the people around me.

3. COMMUNICATING'S HARD, BUT IMPORTANT

Who to ask and how to ask

Communication with your loved ones isn't the only thing that's essential, but also communication with your treating team. Knowing who to ask about sexuality, positioning, care & *safety* is something most of us don't know.

Here's a general summary.

Gynaecologists work with people who have a vulva and/or vagina. Urologists work with those who have a penis. Gastroenterologists and colorectal surgeons work with the digestive system including bowel cancers. Haematologists work with blood and lymphatic cancers. You will also have medical professionals relative to your treatments such as a radiation oncologist for radiotherapy treatments, an endocrinologist for hormone treatments and the effects they have on our bodies and sexuality, and your oncologist who oversees your treatments and chemotherapy. You will have a surgical team relative to the type of procedure you will be having. Psychiatrists are who to speak with regarding mental health and medications, including which medications have which impacts on your sexuality.

All of these people plus your nurses, your doctor or GP (general practitioner if you're in Australia) are all trained to answer your questions.

There are also people like me (OTs) who focus on sexuality, there's pelvic floor physiotherapists and OTs, there are sexologists and sex counsellors as well. You will need to ask; you will need to be your own advocate for your sexuality. But don't worry, if they're not sure how to best answer your question, they will find someone who is. Your care is their priority.

I hear you saying "sure Tess, it's easy to tell us to ask medical professionals questions, but *how* do you ask the questions?" The first step (asking) is the hardest.... But you can do it, I've got your back!

How to say it out loud.

- "What are the precautions I need to take regarding sexual activities during this treatment?"
- "Do I need to avoid sex or do specific things safety-wise? If so, when and for how long?"
- "What do I and my partner/s need to know or do regarding intimate activities?"

- "I'd like to ask a few questions about sex and intimacy during my treatment. Is there a more private space we could go to?"
- "Is there someone I can speak with, who can answer questions about sex during and after treatment?"
- "We/I would like to discuss intimacy during/after treatment. Can we organise a time? And with who?"
- "I'm experiencing some changes with my (insert issue here). Who is the best person to speak to?"
- "How will this treatment affect me/us intimately?"
- "How long after surgery should we wait until it's okay to have sex again? And are there any positions or movements we should avoid?"
- "I'm not sure how to ask this, but I have some questions of a more private nature, who can I speak with about that?"
- "What are the precautions I need to take regarding sexual activities during this type of chemo?"
- "Do I need to avoid sex or do specific things safety-wise during this treatment? If so, when and for how long after the infusion/procedure?"

If a healthcare professional isn't sure or cannot answer your question?

- "Thanks for letting me know, can you please ask someone who might be able to answer?"

- "Okay, can you please tell me who I can ask?"

4. CHEMOTHERAPY

The toxicity of chemotherapy is understandably of concern to those receiving it, but it's okay to be close, intimate and sexual with people on chemo, with a few precautions.

Yes, we need to consider the toxicity of chemo, but there's other things too, such as low white blood cell counts increase risk of infections, and pregnancies can have problems. You may need to wear barriers during sex (including oral sex), or use barriers for specific amounts of time before or after your infusion. By 'barriers' I mean safer sex items like condoms or dental dams (which I discuss more, later in this book).

You may also experience vulvovaginal dryness and discomfort from chemotherapy (I most certainly did). There're reasons why this is common during and after chemo which I'll attempt to explain, but please note, chemotherapy is much more complex than this over-simplification.

Many cancerous cells multiply very quickly, therefore, some chemotherapies are cleverly designed to recognise and attack fast-multiplying cells in the human body. Unfortunately, *some* chemo's can't tell the difference between a fast-multiplying cancer cell, and a fast-multiplying normal healthy cell. Hence the saying "chemo does not discriminate". This is also why on many types of chemo; our hair falls out. Hair follicles are some of the fastest growing (and multiplying) cells in the human body, which the oh-so-indiscriminatory chemo recognises and attacks. You know where else in the body has very fast-multiplying cells that chemo finds? The delightful and protective mucous membranes throughout our body in places like the mouth, stomach, bladder, urethra, vagina and more. Mucous membranes contain fast-growing epithelial cells, so of course the all-seeing chemo recognises and attacks these cells, and the resulting impacts can be mouth-ulcers, stomach ulcers, reflux, UTIs and vaginal dryness and pain. If you're having the type of chemo where a side-effect is hair loss and mouth ulcers, meaning you're having the type of chemo that attacks fast-multiplying cells, having vulvovaginal changes is pretty normal too. If you are suffering from vulvovaginal dryness and pain, please take a look at the mini-book in this series 'A Better Normal for Vaginal Dryness & Pain' for guidance and solutions on how to manage and recover this.

And bringing it back to intimacy and the burning

question "how do you know what precautions you need to follow during chemo?" Ask! As your precautions will differ depending on what chemo type and regime you're on, you'll need to ask your treating team.

Who?

Your oncologist and chemotherapy nurse will 100% know the answers to your questions.

When?

Preferably before you start chemo, but it's never too late to ask (I had these discussions while I was sitting in the chemo chair).

Now here's something very important. If you're someone wanting to have penetrative sex during chemotherapy (vaginally or anally), lubricants are *essential*. Your body will be dehydrated and your tissues may become extra sensitive from this treatment. Lubricants are easily purchased and they really do make things better, however, please use something other than water-based lubricants. They get absorbed into your body like a sponge (as that's what the body does even when it's not dehydrated from chemo), so you need something that will stay slick for longer. I recommend silicone-based lubes Überlube or Sliquid Silver, they're so great. Others use organic coconut oil for lubrication (but can cause thrush with some people, so have caution), or an organic wax-based product Olive & Bee. Lubricants are to me, a safer sex item and worth proper discussion, so later in this book, I cover lubricants in much more detail.

If you experience pain during penetration and you're using lubricants, *stop* and chat with your treating team. For those with a vagina, you may need to use an internal moisturiser to help the tissues rehydrate and become less sensitive. Heal first, play later (refer to the mini-book 'A Better Normal for Vaginal Dryness & Pain' for more on this topic). Penetrative sex should *never* hurt.

Also, your sexual function may change, things may not work as they used to. Maybe your orgasms take longer, maybe they're more or less intense, maybe you don't orgasm anymore, perhaps your erections are changing, you no longer get wet or you simply want sex less. These are common side-effects from chemo and may not be permanent. Remember that your body is processing toxins to treat a disease. You will experience changes in your body, if you're worried, chat with your oncologist or doctor.

I was told before I started chemotherapy that I would need to wear protection to avoid causing my partner "harm", as I would be so toxic. I was petrified of hurting the people around me, I honestly felt like I could damage the people I loved from how 'poisoned' I was. I was scared. I truly regret not asking my chemotherapy nurse for more information about what exactly I needed to be careful of and when. As it wasn't as bad as I thought and from that fear, I withdrew physically from the people around me. So, please learn from my mistakes and ask the nurses/the oncologist for clear guidance.

What do we do?

- Communicate with each other and your oncologist/chemo nurses.

- Be transparent about your side-effects such as pain, fatigue, rashes, changes in sensitivity, pleasure, libido. Tell your date/partner(s) what's going on and how you're doing. Sex can be soft, gentle, and doesn't need to involve penetration. If you're open about how you're doing and what's going on in your body, you can still be intimate around that.

- Use a silicone, wax or oil-based lubricant (see the upcoming 'lube is life' section for more info).

- Explore touch that isn't penetration or orgasm focussed, like the two-minute game (see the 'simple ideas for connecting' section).

- Use barriers if/when needed as advised by your oncologist such as external/internal condoms or dental dams.

- You could shower before and after intimacy to help avoid UTIs.

- Remember, your body not acting normally during chemo is pretty normal!

- For partners: Be gentle, we won't break. Yes, we're sick, but you can totally touch us. Cuddle us, have sex with us, just check in, communicate and remember...don't be afraid of us, be cautious *with* us!

How to say it out loud.

- "What are the precautions I need to take regarding sexual activities during chemo?"

- "Do I need to avoid sex or do specific things safety-wise during chemo? If so, when in my cycle and for how long after the infusion?"

- "Do I need to do anything different sex-wise while I'm taking these chemo tablets?"
- "I'd like to ask a few questions about sex and intimacy during my treatment, is there a more private space we could go to?"
- "I have a few questions about having chemo and if that changes anything sexually, is there someone I can ask?"
- "My partner and I would like to discuss bedroom activities during treatment, can we organise a time? And with who?"
- "Can I have sex during chemotherapy?" (If yes) "Is there anything in particular I need to know regarding safety? Do these precautions include oral sex?"
- "If I do need to wait, how long do I need to wait until after my infusion/taking these tablets?"
- "Is there a resource where I can get this in writing? It's hard for me to remember details".
- "Can you please write this down for me? As I won't remember everything and this is important to know, thank you".

If a healthcare professional isn't sure or cannot answer your question?

- "Thanks for letting me know, can you please ask someone who might be able to answer?"
- "Okay, can you please tell me who I can ask?

Chemotherapy can be quite different for everyone, and our level and intensity of side-effects can vary person to person. I've listed below some other resources available in this series if you are needing specific advice on some of the more particular potential side-effects from chemo.

For further side-effect specific intimacy and sexuality supports chemo may cause, refer to:

- 'A Better Normal for **Vaginal Dryness & Pain**': For people with vulvovaginal pain, dryness, loss of pleasure or if it feels sandpapery and sex hurts.
- 'A Better Normal for **Libido**': For people experiencing drops and changes in their libido/desire.
- 'A Better Normal for **Body Confidence**': Anyone struggling with changes in their body confidence,

lower self-esteem and how to navigate the changes in our body from treatments.

- 'A Better Normal for **Fatigue'**: For people with fatigue, something that can occur during and long after treatments and can greatly impact our sexuality.

- 'A Better Normal for **Changes in Erection**': For people experiencing changes in erection, orgasm and sensitivity.

- 'A Better Normal for **Pain'**: For anyone with pain. Just like fatigue, pain can occur during treatments, but also long after.

- Or if a few of these apply to you, I recommend the all-in-one larger resource **'A Better Normal; Your Guide to Rediscovering Intimacy After Cancer'**, which includes all of the information in the above listed mini-books (and more), conveniently in the one book.

5. CHANGES IN SENSATION

I've been speaking quite generally about how we can rehabilitate our desire and strengthen our pleasure pathways, but I'm going to get a little more specific in this section. In particular, the loss of sensation and erogenous zones through surgeries and/or treatments, and how losing sensation doesn't necessarily mean losing your sexuality.

I had a breast removed and reconstructed from my lower back tissue nearly two years ago and as I type this, still have no nipple. The breast is firm, a different shape, points in a different direction, feels colder to the touch (could be in my mind) and has zero sensation (not in my mind). Initially, I was in my head about it, feeling self-conscious, embarrassed and anxious (especially the one nipple missing part). Losing breast sensation and pleasure is still hard for me. I miss it; I've lost a piece of my sexuality and I hear this from so many others I support, in reference to not only breasts, but other body parts that have been removed or lost sensation from treatments.

The amazing thing about the human body is that we can create *new* erogenous zones! Remember, our sex and pleasure are what's between our ears and not our legs.

If you're experiencing a loss of sensation due to your treatments perhaps damaging the nerves, sensation for some can come back, and sometimes not (depending on the level of damage). But there is hope.

Sensation where nerves are intact is exactly the same as a bicep, which gets stronger the more you exercise it. You can 'create' and 'recreate' highly pleasurable erogenous zones all over (and in) your body, with slow soft touch and being present to how good it feels. In particular, if you're feeling numbness and loss of sensation on or in your genitals, repeated touch and in particular massage can 100% help you regain your sensation and pleasure (refer to the 'Vulva Pleasure Masterclass' and 'Penis Pleasure Masterclass' information in the 'resources' section). If you have loss of sensation due to permanent nerve damage or removal, over time, you can have such amazing pleasure from other areas of your body (neck/inner thighs/ears/lips/belly/lower back etc.). How is this done?

Being intimate, focussing on *slow touch* while being curious can start the rewiring process. It's how we create new erogenous zones and enhance pleasure/sensation that may already be there, but just isn't very strong. If you're wanting to recover sensation and pleasure on/in your genitals, I can't recommend soft penis massage and vulva massage highly enough. Even just twice a week has great outcomes over time.

If you're wanting to recover and improve sensation on your body, play the 2-minute game (described in the next section) asking for attention to other parts of your body, offer yourself soft slow touch when you wake up in the morning for 5 minutes each day or if you need extra support and guidance, my online 'connection & cancer' course (refer 'resources' section). Your inner thighs can be just as erotic as say, your breasts once were with touch.

I've used the same techniques to help people post-stroke regain sensation on their arms, when working in neurological rehabilitation. With a little repetition and attention, you can enhance your pleasure and sensitivity too. Neurological change doesn't happen overnight, but over time it can and does happen.

Remember, pleasure is still pleasurable, even if it's somewhere else on your fabulous body.

In the meantime, brain-chatter from things like self-consciousness, anxiety or stress can be the barrier to enjoying touch on your body and also that rewiring process. If you're getting intimate and feeling self-conscious about your body, pop a little lacy number on, or an item of clothing that's a lovely, sensual material. Something that *feels* nice and helps reduce the anxiety. This will help get your head back into the experience.

It's okay to get sexy while wearing clothing. Or try some positions that aren't so full-frontal to help you relax and enjoy. The key to enhancing your pleasure, to strengthening those sensory and pleasure pathways is to be present, and we can't do that when we're in our heads.

I also want to note that I have a sense of loss, loss of a part of my body which was a source of *so* much pleasure for me. Please allow yourself time to grieve, process and share how you're feeling. None of this is easy, but the loss of a body part, or loss of sensation on an area of your body doesn't have to mean the loss of your sex or your pleasure all together.

Just like everything else in cancer, it's a process and can take time, but speaking from personal experience as someone who has rehabilitated themself through these touch and massage practices, it's well worth it.

6. SIMPLE IDEAS FOR CONNECTING

Something we often do, especially in intimacy, is develop patterns. Intimacy, sex, affection can start to look like the same thing, or doing things in a particular and similar way. In regards to maintaining connection and accessing pleasure during chemo, we need to go slow, maybe change it up so we feel more comfortable and sometimes that's tricky when our relationships and sex look a certain way.

In this section I give you some ways you can have a date-night with someone (or yourself!) which isn't the standard form of what sex might look like to you, but allows you to have fun, connect with yourself, feel good in yourself and feel good with others. The ultimate ideas to keep your sexuality alive and present during chemotherapy. Think of it like keeping the sexual coals burning, so relighting the fire is easier!

The activities I've listed and described are ones I've taught, read about and love to do - and are my top picks for you to try yourself. It's not an exhaustive list, but will give you a start (i.e., trust yourself and you can decide what works for you). Not all will appeal to you, that is fine. They are varied enough so that hopefully there's something for everyone that seems appropriate to try. Remember, these can be done to the level that is right for you, with the person that is right for you. These can be done with a close friend, your carer, by yourself, partners and even family members!

Q&A

I am obsessed with this verbal game and full credit to Roger Butler from Curious Creatures who created it. It's so useful and fun to play if you're in a position where you want to communicate with someone, but it's hard to bring up an awkward topic or start a conversation. It's also great to play any time anywhere, and I love it in social or private settings. It's so simple yet an incredible way to deeply communicate and connect with strangers, loved ones, friends and everyone else. During many of my treatments, I struggled (and still do) to keep up with conversations that involved more than two people as the brain-fog/cancer-brain had my attention span so low. I also struggled at times to have conversations about how I was feeling and where I was at. I often played Q&A as a way to be able to listen to one person at a time, and still have valuable, connective conversations with the people around me. I also play it one-on-one to have meaningful conversations with a partner or friend, while communicating was/is so difficult. Simply put, Q&A makes good conversation great, and when you're struggling, it's a life-saver.

How it works.

Someone asks a question, any question, such as: How was your day? How are you feeling in your body? What do you love about your partner right now? What is your relationship to your sex? Do you like cake more than ice-cream? Anything.

The person sitting to the left of the person who asked the question, answers it first. When they are finished, it goes to the next person to the left, finishing with the person that asked it.

There are a few extra rules:

- Every answer is perfect.
- Every question is perfect.
- No interrupting someone's answer, wait until they have told you they are finished answering, before sharing your thoughts.
- You can 'pass' on a question (or make something

up!).

- You can call 'Tangent' or 'Time' by making a 'T' symbol with your hands. This indicates that someone may be off on a tangent or taking too much time to answer. We always say "thank you" for a 'T'.

- The person who asks the question, always answers it last.

It may seem strange, having a verbal Q&A game in a book about connection and the importance of intimacy, but there's a theme here. Cancer interrupts life, which includes relationships. Medications, treatments, fatigue, nausea, stress, it all interferes and open communication for some can seem too hard. Try this game, try it a few times, it was and still is, a 'go-to' for me, when I want to connect.

Where? You can play it anywhere. Try it in the bath, the couch, at dinner, in the car, a BBQ or a few rounds at the end of the week to see how you're going. It's a beautiful time to be honest, because the rules are that you can't be interrupted and every answer is perfect.

This is also your saving grace if conversations are hard, paying attention is tricky and keeping up with multiple people talking at once. If you let people know what you need and where you're at, they will most likely help you out. I noticed social chatter was a way for people to let me know that 'everything was fine'. But it wasn't, I couldn't concentrate, I couldn't follow the conversation, I quickly forgot what people were saying and I got super stressed. As soon as I mentioned I needed conversation to slow down, that's exactly what happened. Remember, you will need to let people know what you need, and they will be grateful for the guidance. Q&A is a brilliant way to have social structure, and still offer wonderful connections with everyone present.

Little, lovely treats

Sit down and write a list of 5 - 10 things that are small and easy to do, that make you feel special or connected to yourself. Little, lovely treats. If you have a close friend or loved one, get them to do the same, write a list of little lovely things they enjoy. This could be a foot massage, a bath, a favourite wine, a nice cheese with salami and a childhood film (my personal favourite), moisturising each other's hands/backs/necks/chests, looking at photos together, a blindfolded touch experience, a game of loving

Q&A (just described in this section) or dancing to your favourite music.

So, when a time comes, when you're feeling like you would like to connect, be intimate, share affection and don't know what to do? Get the list out and see what you're/you're all in the mood for.

All of these small treats should ideally be things that can be done in your home or very close to where you're staying, and don't take a lot of energy. You want your energy to be spent on connecting and enjoying yourself and others' company, not setting up or travelling to a location.

These 'small treats' lists are your go-to. When you're stuck in your head or having a bad day, get the list out. Soak your feet and moisturise them, do yoga, have a self-pleasure session or pleasure a partner, eat an entire pizza when those taste-buds are back online or get your favourite film and a pot of your favourite tea. The point is that you want an easy way to feel special involving yourself, and possibly those close to you. Simple, sensual, special treats that connect you with yourself/others.

Warming and calming
This small yet intimate task can really let you relax, unwind

and get connected. A gentle, beautiful way to connect with yourself or with someone else, is by enjoying a warm bath. Relaxing in a body of warm water (not too hot!) has so many positive effects on the body. Muscles relax, our nervous system down-regulates (relaxes), it can reduce stress, muscle tension eases, pain can lessen, blood circulation improves, the list goes on. Add a cup of tea, a glass of wine, something playing on a screen you can see or some quality Q&A (again see earlier in this section) if you have a 'bath-buddy' with you.

The waterless bath

Baths not your thing, or you don't have one? I have for you, the waterless bath experience. Pop your electric blanket on a nice low setting or warm up a heat pack on the couch and create a warm snuggly cocoon for yourself or for you and your pet, child, friend or lover. The intent is to create warmth, intimacy, safety and connection - baths are not essential for this, but feeling safe and snuggly is.

A royal bathing

Credit for this idea goes to my primary carer, who 'softens' the daily activities to connect and show love, and has also used this technique when caring for a friend while undergoing treatments for brain cancer (spoiler, they loved it!). Is your partner, lover, friend or carer helping you with your personal care? Such as dressing, washing or even simply helping you dry your feet after the shower? If this is the case, every once in a while, ask the person assisting with your care to take their time with it. Turn it into an almost worshipping, lovingly sensual dressing or bathing. Imagine the treatment someone might get in a luxury ancient Roman spa.

Slowly wash the feet, slowly caress and wash the back, take your time enjoying putting clothing on someone, let the materials softly brush over the skin. Attention and intention are drivers of pleasure and going slowly allows this to happen. Yes, we are often time poor and we go into 'automatic mode', however this is a lovely five-minute task which can be added into daily life quite easily and shows care, love and affection. This small activity acts as a reminder to each other, you're not in a clinical environment, you're not a nurse going through the rounds with a patient, you're caring for someone, someone you care about. Be soft, be gentle, be present. What a treat and what a connector. And it only needs to take an extra five minutes or so.

A simple good night kiss

Life is hectic and a cancer diagnosis doesn't lighten the load. Finances, appointments, family life, medications, symptoms and more, can fill up the days. The only time you may actually see a partner or lover is at the end of the day. If this is you, think about taking five minutes, when you're in bed together getting ready for sleep. Lie down facing each other and look into each other's eyes. Touch noses if you like, hold hands, intertwine feet, hold eye contact, share a good-night statement, breathe together or share a kiss on the lips. It's a time where you're both settling down and both in the same spot, it's a great time to use it to connect.

Don't go to bed at the same time as the person you live/share space with? That's okay, ask that you get 'tucked-in' or tuck your partner in. Get the blankets up to their chin, wish them good night, give them a kiss and a few words of love. It's just such a sweet thing. And if you don't share a house with your loved ones? Sweet, loving good night text messages mean the world!

Self-pleasure

Our entire bodies are capable of pleasure and giving yourself some time, some touch and love is a beautiful way to connect with yourself and get those happy chemicals flowing. During treatments you may be tired, stressed, sore, in pain or feeling flat. Whether you're single or partnered, a lovely way to calm and connect with yourself is to give your body, soft, loving touch. This can, but doesn't necessarily need to involve your genitals or you getting aroused. Our bodies are complicated things and treatments can make our body almost feel like a stranger, so getting to know it again can be wonderful.

Give yourself some time, show yourself you're special and set yourself a date. Be it once a fortnight, once a week, or whenever you feel slightly motivated. It's nice, the first few times if you try to leave genitals out of it, just to see what it's like to focus on your body in a different way. We don't give ourselves enough one-on-one time and this is most definitely the case for personal intimate touch. Be curious, explore, hug yourself, scratch, tap, softly touch the skin, find what your body is and isn't enjoying, what it does and doesn't enjoy at that moment. I'm a firm believer that offering ourselves self-pleasure and understanding our bodies is essential for us to be able to connect with others. Regardless if you're partnered or not, having some time with yourself is healthy, it's calming, and it's connecting.

Massage swaps

This may seem like a strange thing to recommend, but hear me out. Touch, care, love and affection are all things many of us forget about during and after treatments. If you're unsure of what your body wants in an arousal, erotic sense, your immediate fallback plan can be massage. Having someone massage you, gives focus on physical, attentive touch without that pressure of it needing to lead to sex. It's pleasurable, it's intimate and gets you connected (and it feels so good!). Massage swaps can also act as an 'ice-breaker', if you're with a partner or on a date and it's been a while since you've touched each other (which is common). This is a lovely and accessible way to ease back into a physical and touch based dynamic without the pressure to 'perform' or 'be sexy'. If you're not partnered and want some touch, but aren't sure how? There are many very skilled professional massage therapists out there, even the 'pop-in' 10-minute massage parlours have amazing touch and anything that connects you to your body and feels good, is a win.

Another amazing benefit of doing massage swaps, is it's a way for a partner or lover to get used to touching your changed body. So often, I support partners through their fear and anxiety of hurting their partner by touching them. A simple massage can be a way to have your partner touch your body and even start to explore areas they are hesitant to touch (like surgery sites or scars). With a little encouragement, direction and permission from you, these fears and anxieties can be overcome, together.

An undressing ritual

How we see ourselves and also, the fear of being naked in front of another person (and ourselves) is one of the most common concerns I help people with. And chemo can really impact our appearance and in turn, our body and sexual confidence. Undressing rituals are a method of removing clothing for yourself, or another, in a way that is gentle while allowing space for nervousness and shyness, while inviting acceptance and positive regard. You can do this solo by yourself in front of a mirror as a way to get used to your new body, or with a date or partners.

<u>How it works.</u>

There's a lot of scope for variety here so feel free to bend and change this to suit you, but here's the basics. Standing in front of the mirror or someone else, you choose one item of clothing at a time to take off, and as you remove it you make a personal statement. Something that is true, that is how you feel, but also as a way to process, release and move towards acceptance. It's a neat psychological trick and can be wonderful. If you're doing this with a partner, take turns, so after you remove an item of clothing and make a statement, they do the same. Then it's your turn again, and so on.

<u>By statements I mean things like;</u>

- As I remove my shoe, I let go of how hard I am on myself.
- As I take off my shirt, I let go of my self-consciousness.
- Removing my belt is me removing the restrictions of society's ridiculous beauty standards.
- As I remove my bra, I welcome in love and acceptance of my body.
- As I take off my scarf, I release my fear.

- By taking off my pants, I am freeing myself of anxiety.
- By removing my pink sparkly cowboy hat, I am letting go of my tiring day.

Or, if that form of statement doesn't feel right, you could try positive words as you remove clothing and show parts of your body:

- As I look at my arm, I notice the smooth skin I have.
- While looking into the mirror, I'm loving the freckles I have on my face.
- With my chest exposed I feel an appreciation for being alive.
- As I look at my genitals, I notice the awesome curls in my pubic hair.
- As I see my stomach, I see scars/marks of me living, and making it through
- While looking at my lower back, I like the curve where it joins my bottom.

I have done this by myself in front of a mirror, with a long-term partner and also on a date. It was surprisingly effective on the date, as I was very self-conscious about my body and didn't know how to transition from clothed to well, not-clothed. We both took turns slowly removing an item of clothing, we looked into each-other's eyes, we were honest and it was magic. It helped me relax and it helped them understand how I was feeling and how I was struggling.

Go slow. If you're doing this alone in front of the mirror, it can be quite confronting. Don't feel like you need to fully undress, you may need to do this gradually over time. You could remove one additional item of clothing in the mirror to look at and love each time you do this, so it's nice and slow. I've done it several times alone, as a way to slowly look at myself and get used to my changed and abnormal body. I cried a lot, but it truly helped me with body acceptance and processing my grief for the body I used to have. Follow yourself, breathe and trust that you can stop if you need to. If you're with someone and you don't want to get naked, you can remove 'imaginary' items of clothing (like an orange feather boa, a sequin vest, rainbow suspenders etc.) or simply ask to stop. You could also do this with someone, where you take turns in removing an item of clothing off of the other person, while making positive statements about their body. Or maybe you choose the item of clothing on yourself to remove and your partner/date shares statements of love and appreciation of that particular body part. The best part of this activity is that there's room to change this to what feels right for you, at the pace that's right for you.

Chatty-massage

If you're liking the ideas in this book about learning more about what you want and giving more feedback in intimacy and pleasure, but aren't really sure how to do that, this one's for you. 'Chatty massage' is very simple, and is the perfect way to get better at figuring out what you want or don't want, and also, how to ask for it. Plus, this is another excellent activity to do, if your partner is feeling a little hesitant to touch your body, because they're scared of hurting you.

How it works.

Easiest done in pairs, one of you is the 'masseuse', and the other receives the 'massage'. But there's a twist. The person lying down, the one receiving the 'massage' is actually directing the masseuse on what to do. Sounds easy right? Well, there's a little more to it.

The person who is receiving direction, the 'masseuse' is only able to do exactly that, receive and follow directions. They cannot take over the experience or offer what they *think* the person receiving might enjoy. They can only follow the directions given by the person lying down who is 'receiving' the massage. Most importantly however, is that if the masseuse/person following directions doesn't hear something along the lines of "keep going" or "I like this continue please" or a new instruction, they must stop touching the person giving the directions all together by gently removing their hands and waiting for the next instruction.

Why does the person have to stop touching after 10 seconds of silence you ask? For the person who is receiving the directions, this is a lesson in being guided in touch, in taking feedback and more importantly, not making assumptions as to what the other person may want and 'winging it'. For the person receiving the massage/giving directions, it allows them to learn how to ask for what they'd like and how to communicate if they'd like something to stop, continue or to change. It's powerful stuff. It's also an incredible way for them to really explore their body and to learn what they do and don't like at the pace that's right for them.

Giving feedback and knowing how to receive it during intimacy is the thing that makes a good time, a great time. But we're not taught how to talk about sex or our bodies. We're definitely not taught how to explore our likes and dislikes in a safe and compassionate way. The world would be better if we were. Chatty massage (as simple as it seems) is your way to flex those communication muscles and learn so much about your and your partner's pleasure.

If you're not sure where to start, try doing it together sitting on the couch and just on the hand or shoulders to start with. Or have a clothes-on play together while you get used to how it works. You could even set a timer so you have 5 or 10 minutes each of giving and receiving while you're trying it out. You can start by exploring things like soft touch on your arms, maybe scratchy touch on your back, massage touch on your neck and thighs. Soft kisses on your lower back. Feel free to get creative as the person following directions is going to stop if you don't ask for it to keep going, or ask for something to change. This is the safety mechanism, so you both can feel free to relax and have a bit of fun with it.

You may be thinking that the more difficult role in

this, is that of the person who's lying down and giving the directions. Funnily enough, when I work with partners together and I teach them this activity it's the complete opposite. It's the person receiving directions and having to stop and withdraw touch after 10 seconds of silence that struggles the most! Due to this, I'm going to repeat the rule as it's surprisingly tough for people, but is so important. If the 'masseuse' doesn't hear a direction after 10 seconds, they must stop what they're doing, remove their hands and wait. This is what will help the person giving direction do exactly that, as they will *have* to give you direction when you stop. So much of our intimacy is guess-work and with the impacts of cancer treatments, clarity and communication could never be more important. Stopping the touch after a short amount of time is a way to help each other practice giving and receiving feedback and most importantly, tuning in to what you do and don't want at the time.

It will 100% feel clunky and awkward at first, just like everything else we try in life for the first time. Don't worry too much about it as this is play, and yes play can be clunky, but it can also be fun. Have a laugh and have another go. Communication is the number one sex move, and this activity is the perfect way to practice.

The two-minute game

Finally we learn about the two-minute game!!!! Life coach Harry Faddis created the 'three-minute game' and I was taught the 'two-minute game' from Roger Butler at Curious Creatures, and it's simply brilliant. This game is suitable for those experiencing treatment and their loved ones, is great when you have no idea how to connect with someone or where to start and is a wonderful way to gently get to know each other's bodies again.

Here's the rules.

- Set a timer or an alarm on your phone for two minutes.
- Pick who goes first, then that person asks for something they would like for 2 minutes (some examples are listed shortly).
- If you all agree, start the timer and give the person whatever they asked for.
- When the timer goes off, completely stop what you're doing.
- Then it's the next person's turn to ask for something they would like for two minutes.

- If everyone agrees, start the timer and go.

- Once the timer goes off, again, stop what you're doing.

- And repeat.

That's it. Really, that is the game. So simple, yet so effective. You can play it for as long as you like - 10 minutes or an hour, or however long you have energy and are having fun. Time can really fly when playing this game.

Also, this game can be played with anyone, not just someone you're in a relationship with. It could be a friend, family member, carer and doesn't have to be in pairs. There are so many ways to connect, to touch and be touched, which this game can help you discover.

One of the first (out of possibly hundreds) times I played this, I wasn't sure what to ask for. So, of course, I asked for a shoulder massage. Then, that became a slow back scratch. Then full body soft touch and I was amazed at how starting simply and being left wanting more (thanks to that timer) guided me to what I would like next. Asking for what you want can be difficult at first, but this game allows you to develop that skill with practice. Asking for what we want is such an essential skill to have during cancer treatments (and always).

A common question when introducing the two-minute game in workshops is, "what happens if someone asks for something you don't want to do?" Say "no-thank you" with a smile and discuss an alternative (such as touching the chest or back rather than genitals). It's okay. Wait, it's more than okay, it's wonderful to say 'no'. Saying what we don't want is equally (maybe more) important than saying what we do want. The goal is to find that optimal place where everyone is happy giving and receiving.

Here's a few reasons why this game can work for you:
Our genitals aren't always up for being played with, so when it's your two minutes, ask for something that doesn't include them (you have your whole body).

This game can allow connection, even with different levels of libido. Someone might want sexual touch for two minutes and if you're happy to give it, great! Your two minutes could be something that suits your mood such as "tell me your favourite joke using your hand as a puppet". The possibilities are endless and you can ask for exactly what you want, while easily avoiding what you don't want.

Bodies impacted by treatment can change dramatically and unpredictably, be it sensation, arousal, pain, surgical sites etc. This game allows you to relearn how your body works or doesn't work (where those desensitised parts are, where it's sore, where it's pleasurable, how toys or lubes feel).

If you're playing this with a partner and are worried about where things may lead to? Take 'typical' sex off the table for the entire game. You could have a 'no genital contact' rule or even leave your clothes on. Remove the pressure to perform or get aroused. Obligation & expectation are the enemy of arousal, feeling safe and relaxed is its catalyst. Get creative, enjoy yourselves without that pressure. You can enjoy pleasure from soft intimate touch anywhere on the body.

The two-minute game has many communication benefits and can act as a gentle ice breaker. With changed sexuality and changed intimacy (with or without illness), can come distance and avoidance. Talking about sex is not easy, especially when things are different. This game gently offers a way to help navigate those tricky feelings while also acknowledging the elephant in the room. While we're at it, let's erase any feelings of 'being selfish' or 'a taker'. Asking for your neck to be gently kissed for two minutes, or to be told why this person loves you for two minutes, is simply playing the game. It can seem difficult, but remember, you have to ask, it's the rules! Through my work as a sexuality and consent workshop facilitator, I'm always shocked at how many people tell me that they have never asked for what they want before. Practice makes perfect and it does get easier the more you do it.

Here's a list of things you could ask for, for your two minutes:

- Can you please lower the lights, put some relaxing music on that I would like, bring me water and join me on the couch in two minutes?
- Hold my hand and tell me how you're doing for two minutes.
- Massage my (insert body part here) for two minutes.
- Starting at my neck, ever so softly touch my entire body, back to feet over two minutes.
- Tell me about your day through interpretive dance.
- Put on a song and show me your silliest/favourite dance move.
- Make me a cup of tea in two minutes.
- I would like to cuddle for two minutes.

- I would like to offer you a shoulder massage for two minutes (that's still your two minutes, but if you're not up for being touched, you can touch others. It's all about what YOU want).
- Massage my head.
- I would like to stroke your hair with your head in my lap.
- Lightly touch my beautiful bald head for 2 minutes.
- Gently kiss my neck/chest/thighs/back for two minutes.
- Show me how you like to be kissed, for two minutes.
- Kiss my face and tell me things you love about me for two minutes.
- Softly breathe on my entire body, ending with my genitals for two minutes (YUM!).

If you're thinking, "ugh, whatever Tess. Some of us don't know how to just simply know what you want and ask for it." You're right, I hear you. None of us are taught this, but I have a solution for you. A beautiful baby-step towards the 2-minute game and flexing those 'asking' muscles, is by playing the previous activity 'chatty massage'.

Active receiving

'Active receiving' is a way to connect with a lover/partner to the level that is right for you, when you're not feeling sexy or like having sex and maybe need a little bit more time to get those feelings flowing.

It's a one-way touch experience, and a great way to enjoy touch. I'll explain a little more. There are many expectations and misconceptions in intimate activities, and a super common one is that it should always be a two-way experience. You give and receive pleasure at the same time. Well, this doesn't necessarily always have to be the case, and I offer you a wonderful way to connect in a one-way touch format, very similar to 'chatty massage' mentioned previously. This is wonderful for people with mismatched libido, delayed arousal responses, if someone is not wanting to receive intimate touch or may not know what they want at that moment, but would love to see a partner have pleasure and enjoy themselves.

How it works.

Someone lies/sits down (or is in any comfortable position), asks for what type of touch they want, and constantly directs that person in how they touch them. The other person does exactly what they are being told to do. That's it! It's incredibly fun and accessible.

Imagine the person giving the touch and receiving the directions has no mind of their own, they are an inanimate object that only responds to commands. For the person following instructions, it can free you from that common brain chatter ("am I doing this right? Are they enjoying this? Are they pretending?"), as you're just doing what you're told.

Some examples of directions the person who is receiving touch (and giving all directions) could give are: "Massage my shoulders. Can you now scratch my back? Yum, thanks, can you go slower and a bit firmer? Softly touch my body up and down, neck to feet with your fingertips and don't stop until I say. Now, lightly pinch my inner thighs. Breathe cool breath on my nipples." Anything you want, just ask.

Unlike in chatty massage where the person following directions stops all together if they don't hear anything after a short while, in 'Active Receiving', the person giving the touch can check in to see if it's how the receiver wants it ("How is this pressure? Would you like me to move my hands faster or slower?") *without* stopping. The person following directions doesn't change anything, doesn't alter any style without being directed. If the person giving touch doesn't receive any directions for a while and isn't sure if this is still what the person receiving still wants? Keep doing what you were last asked to do and ask the question "how could you enjoy this more?"

Similar to chatty massage, this is an incredible skill to learn in the bedroom. Giving directions, asking for what we want, checking in with a lover to get feedback on their level of enjoyment, communicating your desires, all of this leads to better communication and better sex. If you get tired? Simply stop the activity whenever one of you wants. The goal is to enjoy receiving and to enjoy giving. 1 minute, 10 minutes, 20 minutes, it's all perfect.

If you're unsure, give it a go, clothes on, on the couch, using just an arm or hand. Practice following directions, practice giving directions, practice checking in and identifying what you want. There is no goal here, just to have a touch experience, to give or receive pleasure, and enjoy connecting with a partner. It may feel clunky at first, but with practice it flows very easily and you will be amazed at how much you learn about your partner and their body (and yours!).

If this sounds like fun to you, but asking for what you want and giving directions seems a bit daunting, or taking directions and not being the one driving the experience sounds tough, I recommend playing 'chatty massage' or the '2-minute game' a few times first, before jumping into this activity. I say this because it won't be enjoyable if you're still getting used to these styles of intimate communication. Those two activities are wonderful ways to develop these amazingly sexy skills.

7. UH-OH, WHERE'S MY O? (CHANGES IN ORGASM)

Something not often spoken about is how during and after chemotherapy, is that your orgasms/climaxes can change, or sometimes even disappear. I've touched on this briefly; however, this can occur with other treatments too. This is common (it happened to me and many others I support), this is normal, you are normal.

How can they change, you ask? Maybe they're less 'intense', maybe they're more intense. Perhaps you need a lot more time and play (yum!) to 'get there', maybe your body shakes and does the things it normally does, but you don't really feel any actual orgasm. What I call a *'ghost-gasm'*, and was very strange to me during chemo when I first experienced this. There is also the possibility that orgasms and climaxes may not be possible for a while. Sex can still be very pleasurable during cancer treatments, but sometimes our medications block that 'peak-climactic' experience.

Thanks to the wonders of neuroscience, we now know that our body can 100% relearn how to have them, or have *different* ones.

Firstly, know that there are multiple potential blockers to climaxing. If you're on particular antidepressants or undergoing hormone treatments, maybe had nerve damage from surgeries and other things, climaxing (orgasms) may not be achievable just yet. It's okay, you can still have a *lot* of pleasure. Sex can still be great sex during and after cancer, without the end point, without that 'goal'.

If you would like to relearn how to have orgasms, or better put, if you would like to rewire your pleasure so the body you now have can have climaxes (even if they're a little different) here's something to try.

Regular self-pleasure with a few rules

I'm talking even just 2-5 minutes a day (10 would be better).

1. Remove the goal, remove the pressure

Ban the orgasm. You heard me! You're only allowed to touch and enjoy your body to rewire your brain and associate touch with *'goal-free'* pleasure. This neurologically starts to rewire your brain in the background that intimacy isn't about the pressure of that goal. This creates freedom and can be a major stepping stone to your pleasure and orgasm recovery. Better yet, if you have a partner/s, have a 'no orgasm allowed' touch-fest a few times a week. Even if you currently can't orgasm, removing it verbally anyway allows you to enjoy the touch you're receiving (without the guilt, pressure and frustration). Remember, removing the goal can help you get to the goal. You can do this with a partner, but if so, put a timer on and you're only allowed to touch while the timer (5-10mins) is on. It's another way to remove that expectation of it having to 'go somewhere'.

2. Don't forget to breathe.

Breath is powerful, as it not only can be used to down or up-regulate our nervous system, but it also aids in circulating blood to our internal tissues. So many of us tense up and hold our breath when we're in pleasure or when we're *trying* to have an intense moment. It's like we're forcing an orgasm to arrive, which is going to get in the way of you having one! It's like trying to force yourself to go to sleep, the effort of forcing and trying, counteracts where you want to actually go.

Next time you're having pleasure (with yourself or another), relax your muscles and slow down your breath. Remember, this is about pleasure not orgasms, so be curious. Relaxing your body and making sure you're breathing gets blood flow to the deep internal tissues. With blood flow, the tissues get oxygenated and guess what? Our sensitivity increases and so does our pleasure!

If you notice you're tense and/or hold your breath in pleasure, have a few practice runs with yourself. Touch your body, experience pleasure and arousal, but when you notice your muscles tensing up or you're holding your breath, stop, slow down, and only continue when you're relaxed again. Think of it like a pleasure meditation. It can feel strange, but trust me, blood-flow is the key to arousal and pleasure, and we can't circulate blood without breath, and blood can't reach our internal pleasure structures without those muscles being relaxed.

3. Slow it down.

Some of my work includes masturbation coaching with clients, teaching people that there's more than just fast-paced standard movements. When we rush, we get distracted and then that *'should'* brain (the obligation and pressure of getting somewhere) can get in the way. Plus, as just mentioned, going slow allows blood circulation and muscles to relax... again, blood-flow increases our sensation, arousal and our pleasure. Cancer treatments often give us a slower arousal response, so we need more time to really get into it? Orgasms may be achievable; they just need more time and 'warm-up'. If this is you, take a look at the 'toys' section a little later, I have some suggestions for you.

4. Massage

A number one way to recover orgasm is through genital massage (refer to the 'Vulva Pleasure Masterclass' and 'Penis Pleasure Masterclass' in the 'resources' section at the end). We all love massage, it's relaxing, allows our muscles to relax and can reduce tightness while increasing blood-flow. Vulvovaginal and penis massage (preferably soft penis massage) are incredible for orgasm recovery on many levels. Through various massage techniques you can recover and discover new pleasure zones and enhance sensitivity.

5. Repetition.

To make change neurologically you need time and repetition. Self-pleasure and/or massage regularly. A few times a week, over months, maybe 5 mins of loving touch every day if you can (but a few times a week if that's more doable for you). Pleasure rewiring is not a quick fix, but from someone who's been-there-done-that after treatments, it can be done!

6. Exercise.

Exercise helps with arousal as it gets blood-flow to the deeper pelvis structures, engorging tissues and heightening sensitivity. If you can find even just 10 minutes to go for a quick walk or jog, or do some yoga before a pleasure session, this can help increase your sensitivity and arousal, helping pave the way towards orgasms.

7. Lastly, TOYS.

Explore with vibration as it offers stimulation to the deeper tissues and in a way we can't offer naturally. It's a great kick-starter for those times when you want to experience pleasure, but aren't sure exactly what your body enjoys.

Firstly, for people with a vulva, the vagina is not designed to have peak orgasmic experiences, the clitoris is. And although most of our clitoral structure is inside us, we do have a portion of it externally/on the outside of our body for easy access. So, you could try stimulating the head of your clitoris (the part of the clitoris you can touch on the outside of your body) before and during play as a way to warm-up and kick-start your reactive arousal. If your hands don't feel like they're offering you enough sensation, try a 'clitoral vibrator'.

For people with a penis, there are now incredible ranges of vibrators for you. Plus, if you're experiencing changes in erection, know that your delightful soft penis is 100% capable of pleasure and orgasms.

Finally, please know there is nothing wrong with using toys. Just like we use glasses to read better, we can use toys to pleasure better. And toy shopping with a partner? Best foreplay ever!

A quick note, that there are some countries which legally sell THC and cannabis products and some folks tell me that specific strains can influence arousal and their ability to climax. I cannot make recommendations as unfortunately Australia is a little behind and it's not legal here, so I can't access this product. I feel it would be irresponsible of me not to mention this, for those who live in countries and specific states of the US that can access this, and may want to look into it further.

This is very general advice and I know our bodies are

much more complicated than a few simple steps, but the information here is truly powerful. Our desire and arousal are so complicated during and after cancer treatments, and also for partners. Be kind to yourselves, this is tough and the changes in your body may well be temporary.

8.   SEXUAL POSITIONS, TECHNIQUES & TOOLS

Sex as a functional activity is extremely adaptable, with so many possible positions we can put our bodies in and so many adaptations to suit our needs. Here, I offer some suggestions and ways to alter the positions of your body to get around a few of the trickier side-effects of treatments.

Explore, experiment, but make sure you do it from a place of communication and curiosity. You all want to be comfortable and, most importantly, safe, so have a chat beforehand with your lover. Treat it like a brainstorm, note what parts of your body are sore or might need support and figure out how to work around them comfortably and safely. It mightn't seem 'sexy' at first, but these conversations will get easier, and it will make things *much* better. And remember, if it's good, you'll want it more.

DISCLAIMER: These positions are to be used as a guide, not direct clinical recommendations. Please consult your treating team regarding precautions and care relative to your body, and feel into what is right for you, before trying something new. Remember, ask your medical team about any physical restrictions or limitations you may have during and after treatments relative to your symptoms and situation, especially after surgeries. We're all different and only your healthcare team can give you advice specific to you.

And finally, let your pain be your guide, and stop as soon as you feel any discomfort.

Positions for nausea

Having your head above your heart can be relieving, or at least, not make nausea worse. Sexual positions that involve someone sitting up or leaning against something and standing are recommended. Sitting on the couch raised on cushions, standing and bracing yourself while you lean over on a kitchen bench/chest of drawers for stability. For oral sex, standing/leaning back into the corner of a room while the other person kneels on the floor in front of you can work well, as the two corners act as a brace on each side of you. This allows you to worry less about keeping still, and enjoy what is happening more. Try timing things around when your anti-nausea meds are working their best or even having a snack on some bland foods before getting intimate, to help settle your stomach.

Positions for fatigue, lack of energy & oxygen users

The idea of being intimate with someone when your mind and body is fatigued can seem bewildering. Finding a position that doesn't need too much energy is very important. If you're using oxygen, not using too much energy is a way to avoid losing your breath. Sex can be soft, slow, gentle and warm (and still be hot). You don't have to have a full body work-out to have a beautiful connection. Let someone else do the work.

If you are struggling with fatigue (take a look at the mini-book in this series 'A Better Normal for Fatigue' for specific solutions), I recommend keeping a fatigue diary. It comes in handy, to find those times during the day/week/treatment cycles where you have more and less energy. We want to use your energy for pleasure, not for chores! Essentially, you'd want to position the person using oxygen or who is fatigued, in a position that doesn't involve much muscle engagement or movement. Lying on your back, lying on the side or sitting up with your back propped up on a couch or in bed against the wall can involve very little movement and still be intimate.

Being on all fours and having someone behind you can also be done with little energy spent by the person 'receiving'. Stack some pillows on top of each other and pop them under the person's chest so they are still on their knees, but resting on the pillows, rather than holding themselves up. You could even try leaning on or bending over some furniture, while someone can access your yummy behind. These positions are very handy if the other person with you is able to do most of the energetic work, but remember, sex doesn't have to be an Olympic sport to be enjoyable. If both people have low energy, the side-lying position can be great, like a snuggly spoon position.

A wonderful oral sex position, if both people need to use as little energy as possible, or are wheelchair users, is with both lying down. How it works is someone lies on the bed on their side, with knees together and bent towards the chest exposing their genitals, like a fetal or right-angle position. The other person can then lie down on their side and their face can easily access the other person's genitals, both people are lying down and using a lot less energy than other oral sex positions. You can also try a '69' position, but lying on your sides. Imagine a 'lazy-69'.

Plus, hot OT tip here. The more supported and still you are, the less energy you use, so propping yourself up with cushions/leaning against things uses less energy than holding yourself up, and gives you more energy for the fun-stuff.

It's important to note, bodies are complicated and what might work one day, might not the next. It's okay, it's normal, but you need to communicate how you're doing during and after sex. Telling your lover that you're needing to change position because the sheet is rubbing on your chemo rash, or that your muscles are starting to get tired, that you need to slow down due to a bit of nausea, or perhaps a drain tube is getting bumped, is important for both of your enjoyment. Comments like this, are you being great at sex. Make the adjustments you need, see if everyone is doing okay, keep going if you're all comfortable and check in after.

If you want to stop, then stop. Remember, don't force it, don't put up with pain, self-pleasure is always there for a partner if someone wants to continue. Hey, if you stop sex as it's a bit too difficult or is no longer pleasurable and your lover wants to continue pleasure through touching themselves? Offer them a hand!

Key positional tricks.

- The more still and supported you are, the less energy you use.

- Having your chest exposed (not against something or someone) can make it easier to breathe.

- Sitting up, and being still is great for people using oxygen and for nausea.

- Having your chest open and staying upright can be more comfortable if you're experiencing acid reflux.

- A pillow/cushion between the knees separates the thighs and prevents them rubbing together if you have sensitive skin there or a catheter taped to your inner thigh.

- If you're standing up and playing with someone lying on a bed/chair, whether they're on their front or back, you can put some pillows underneath them to raise their pelvis to match the height of yours. This avoids you needing to bend/squat down, which could be tiring or cause joint pain. This is also a great tip if you're playing with or penetrating an anus.

- Empty your stoma pouch/urine collection device before sex and while you're getting used to it. Try positions that leave space around that area such as standing, sitting, lying on your side, being behind someone, or on top of someone.

- If you have tubes or surgery sites, don't lie on them, use cushions to protect them and lie on your other side (your 'unaffected' side) to avoid pushing/putting weight on them.

- Standing or sitting in a corner has more stability than leaning against a flat wall.

- If you're having sex and are using a manual wheelchair? Double check the breaks are on!

- With any wheelchair play, pop the armrests up/take them off if able, it frees up a *lot* of space.

- For wheelchairs that have a tilt-in-space function, this can be great for in-chair partner play!

- If you're uncomfortable deep inside? Use an 'Ohnut' to reduce the depth of penetration.

- Sore joints? Have a bath beforehand or a warm shower and get straight into a warm cosy bed.

- A pillow under your hips raises the pelvis, allowing easier access to the genitals/anus and also supports the lower back.

- A pillow between the thighs can be wonderful for hip & knee joint pain.

- If you find a good position, but it's hard to hold yourself in it? Prop yourself up with cushions or pillows.
- Concerns about continence if you get excited? Having sex in the shower rinses away any urine or faeces that might come out. Avoid using plastic bed sheets as they don't absorb anything and can create more mess. You can pop a towel down on the bed, plus there are great absorbent mats designed for children that wet the bed. I have a 'Squirt Blanket' from Yoni Pleasure Palace, it's machine washable and it's the best.
- Use lubricants, always and forever.
- Get comfy, put cushions under any knees or bums if you're on the ground.
- Lastly, and most importantly, communicate before, during and after about how you're doing.

How to say it out loud.

- "Can we please pause for a second? I just need to re-adjust these cushions, thanks!"

- "I'd love to keep going, but we may need to brainstorm a new position as I'm a bit nauseous/tired/out of breath/sore…"
- "I'm really loving this, could we slow down a bit? I'm losing my breath."
- "This is so great, but I'm having a hot flush, can we sit up so I'm not in so much contact with the bed?"
- "I'm really enjoying this; I just need to top up the lube."
- "It's wonderful to connect with you, but I'm starting to feel a little dry, can you pass the lube please?"
- "Pause, lube top-up!"
- "I'm feeling some discomfort/changes in my erection, how do you feel about some pleasuring with my hands?"
- "I may need to stop; would you like to continue with self-pleasure? Would you like me to touch your body while you pleasure yourself?"
- "Can we please pause? I'm feeling a bit odd and need a moment, thank you."
- "I don't want to keep going as we are, but really want to continue being intimate with you. Is there

some form of different touch or pleasure you might enjoy that I can offer you?"

- "How could you/we enjoy this more?"
- "Is there a speed or pressure of touch that you might enjoy more?"
- "How could this be even better for both of us?"
- "I just wanted to check in, are you comfortable?"
- "Please let me know if you need to change positions at any time."
- "Please call out for more lube if/when you need, it's within arm's reach."
- "I'm loving connecting with you, I just want to make sure you're comfortable?"
- "I know I'm not moving much, but I'm really enjoying this and I'd like to keep going."

Communicating after intimacy (aftercare).

- "Thank you so much, that was wonderful. Is there anything you need or would like in this moment?"
- "Can we please cuddle for a while? I'd like to stay connected with you for a bit longer."
- "I'd love to know what you enjoyed about that experience, and I'll share the same."

- "I'd love to know if there was anything you might like to do differently next time, or explore more, and I'll share the same."
- "Can we lie here together while I catch my breath?"
- "This has brought up a few emotions, I'm okay, but chatting for a short while would be lovely."

9.   LUBE IS LIFE (& OTHER SAFETY ITEMS)

I want to march the streets of every major city across the globe, with thousands of chanting companions screaming for the use of lube. Lubricants are one of the most important and most underused sexual aids and are essential during chemo. Lube is your lovely friend, the friend that is easily and readily available any time you need it. It makes you feel comfortable and safe, and helps you feel good.

I hear some of you say, "But I've never had to use lubricant before. It's never been *needed*," or, "I get my partner/s aroused enough, thanks". Lubricant isn't about mimicking or replacing arousal, it doesn't mean you're doing something wrong; it means you're doing something right. Regardless of your age or your body, lubricant can enhance sexual activity, make it feel better, help it last longer and help make it safer. If sex is toast, lube is the spread. It's a bit like how food tastes good, but add a bit of salt or seasoning and suddenly it's so much better. Some of you might be thinking, "I've always used lube, it's awesome." That's great, keep going!

So, what are they, really? Lubricants are a viscous

(slippery) liquid used to reduce friction when two surfaces rub against each other. If you rub your two hands together, fast, right now, you'll hear the sound of the skin rubbing and your hands will get warm (friction does that). Now, put some lube on your hands, maybe some soap and water and rub your hands together again...it's smoother and nicer, isn't it? That's what lubes do, make two surfaces slippery. Lubricants increase comfort, pleasure and safety, as it protects your delicate genital and anal tissues. What's more important than our safety?

Safety can mean many things. For anuses, penises or vaginas that are dry or sore, lubricants create extra moisture to relieve friction. Reducing friction and smoothing out surfaces can also *enhance* sensation, it protects barriers like condoms and dams, and most importantly, the moisture helps protect the skin from tearing. Skin tears can be uncomfortable, painful, decrease pleasure and also increase infection risk. Lubricants also reduce the risk of condoms breaking (whether on an object or genitals) as a dry environment can pull/rub on the barrier and strain it, or even tear it. Lubricants contribute to a safer sexual experience, and allow you to relax and enjoy more. If you're using lubricants and you're still feeling discomfort, please speak with your treating team and if you have a vulva & vagina, take a look at the book in this series 'A Better Normal for Vaginal Dryness & Pain'.

If it goes in, put it on

The simple rule with lube is this: If anything is going to be inserted anywhere? Make sure it's clean, covered, and use lube. This includes tampons if you're feeling sore, tight or dry. Lube is nothing to be ashamed of or embarrassed about. Have it on your bedside table loud and proud, it shows you care about your and your lovers' well-being.

In Australia you can buy lubricants at your supermarket, local chemist, corner store and petrol station. If you don't want to buy lubricant in person, not a problem. They are easily purchased online and you can order small tubes/small amounts when you're first finding what you like, to avoid breaking the budget. Plus, online stores have more variety and much better quality than what you generally find in your local shop. Lubricants aren't expensive, so you can try many types to work out which ones you like as it makes a big difference to get a lubricant that suits you.

You can get everything from really basic to super

organic to extremely fancy. It's about finding what suits you best, but I'll say this. Lubricants are like aeroplane tickets; you get what you pay for. It can be worth spending a little more for a better experience, especially if you have sensitive skin or atrophy, as the cheaper items may have more chemicals in them and cause a reaction.

What's out there?

There's quite a few different types of lubricants and moisturisers, and it can seem a bit daunting. Don't worry, I've broken it down, so you can find what's good for you.

Water-based:

In Australia you can get these everywhere, and are usable on toys and latex condoms. Water-based lubricants are easily absorbed by our bodies, so it's normal if you need to keep applying. Plus, if you like it very runny, you can also add more water to a water-based lube. Please don't think there is anything wrong if you need to keep adding more during play, it simply means your body is doing what it's designed to do, absorb water. When it comes to water-based lubricants, more is more. And you will constantly need more.

Silicone based:

These lubricants are perfectly safe and are longer lasting, so you don't have to reapply as often as water-based lubes, plus they feel wonderful. Something most silicone lubes are not good for is to use them with silicone toys as it can damage the toy over time. If you're not sure, go to the website of the particular brand you're interested in to see if they specify it's safe to use on a silicone toy or not. Generally found in the FAQ section if their website has one. Toys made of other materials such as stainless steel, rubber, vinyl or glass are fine with this type of lube. If you want to use a silicone toy with your silicone lube, simply pop a condom over the toy creating a barrier between the two. If choosing is a bit overwhelming, I use Überlube and Sliquid Silver, they're so great.

Hybrid:

This means water-based mixed with silicone, it's a 'hybrid' of the two main types of lubricants out there. These lubes last longer than solely water-based lubes as they're mixed, however they still do get absorbed by the body over time, as there is high water content.

Oil-based:

Oil based lubricants such as organic coconut oil or organic castor oil and more, are used by some and certainly work as a lubricant skin-to-skin, however there are a few things to mention. Oil-based lubricants can break down some latex materials which means that it's best to avoid oil-based lubricants when barriers (like latex condoms) are being used. You can buy condoms that are made out of other materials than latex, which are fine with oil-based products. Also, for those who have a vagina, oil-based lubricants can be thicker and harder for the internal tissues to flush out. I know many people who use organic coconut oil as a lubricant (and is great for massage oil), but have caution as it can cause thrush in some. A way to test this is to put a dab of oil on your inner thigh/outer labia to look for any reactions first.

Wax-based:

I'm referring to a particular product here because wax-based lubes aren't a huge thing (yet), but a pelvic floor physiotherapist created an 'intimate cream' made from beeswax and olive oil called 'olive & bee'. As described in the vaginal atrophy section, it can be used as a lubricant and also as an internal moisturiser. I have a few favourite lubes and moisturisers I like to use and this is in my top three. I use it as both a lubricant and a moisturiser. The beeswax is thick and creates a protective barrier, the olive oil has healing properties and because it's so thick and slick, it's pretty great for people with vulva & vaginal atrophy (hence why I love it so much). If you're UTI prone, try it out with caution as it's a thick product and can take the vagina a little extra time to flush any remnants out.

Sterile lubricants:

Generally, water-based, sterile lubes are commonly used in hospitals and clinical settings. It's as the name sounds, sterile. With a lower infection risk, this lube is used by medical professionals and is excellent to use with toys, especially toys/items that will penetrate. Remember me mentioning our very delicate internal tissues? Sterile lubricants can offer that extra layer of safety in case of any tissue damage. They are easily purchased online from medical stores and some online sex stores also. Plus, if you're UTI prone, sterile lubricants can be great as they have such a lower infection risk.

Chemicals:

Avoiding lubricants with high chemical content is recommended. So, don't purchase lubes that are coloured, scented or flavoured. Also, check the ingredient listing on the product label for parabens or other chemically sounding things, as they can irritate the skin. Essentially, if you're reading the ingredients list and you see a word so long you want to buy a vowel in order to be able to read it…..I'd give that word a good old google before buying the product. There are also 100% natural organic options which are easily found online. I've recently discovered lubricants containing colloidal silver, which has anti-inflammatory properties, can reduce itching and burning, promotes healing and doesn't disturb the oh-so-important natural pH levels inside us. This is a very gentle product, so again, if you're someone with discomfort or dryness (pretty common with chemotherapy), this could be a great one to try.

Lubricants used for anal-play:

For anal penetration, it's recommended by many in the industry to use thicker, more viscous lubricants (avoid lubricants with glycerin as they can get sticky and create friction). As a very important job of the rectum is to absorb water, silicone-based lubricants can be great for the anus as there is less water in them, so they last longer. There are also water-based lubricants which are thicker and specially designed for anal play, these are also great, but you *must* make sure they specify they are for anal use. Remember, a standard water-based lubricant will be absorbed quickly into your body and you may experience friction if you don't top up regularly. Whether you're on treatments or not, lubricants are essential as our anuses don't produce moisture on their own, so lubricant makes everything more comfortable. The tissues are quite delicate in there, so if you warm-up your anus (a bit of foreplay doesn't hurt anyone - literally!) and use lubricants, you will avoid causing any damage. As I keep saying, the anus is a highly pleasurable area of the human body and it needs care before being played with.

Vaginal moisturisers:
As discussed previously in the 'our poor vajootz' section, internal moisturisers are exactly what they sound like. A moisturiser that gets applied internally inside the vagina, repeatedly over a period of time. Some are only accessible

via a script from your oncologist which may contain hormones and others are available at pharmacies on the shelf. Please ask your doctor before purchasing one and speak with the pharmacist when you're there, about the medications/chemo you're on. There may be ingredients that will cause a reaction to your internal tissues, the only way to know if something could benefit you, is to consult with your treating team.

Some vaginal moisturisers have hormones such as oestrogen or testosterone in them, so if your cancer is hormone receptive, this may have negative impacts. It may be fine, but better to be sure and safe. Other internal moisturisers mimic a steroid 'prasterone' that our body naturally produces in our adrenal glands (commonly sold as 'intrarosa'), which depending on your cancer type and treatment, may not be safe to use. You will need to speak to your oncologist to ask if a vaginal moisturiser is appropriate for you to use and they will recommend what is best for you.

There are hormone free moisturisers on the chemist and pharmacy shelves, some need prescriptions from doctors, and others you can order online. If you need a hormone free internal moisturiser, look for anything that contains hyaluronic acid. It's a slick substance we produce naturally in our bodies to keep our synovial joints moving smoothly and it's great for our internal tissues.

There are also moisturisers which can be used externally, for the vulva area. Again, you will need to consult your treating team to see what is recommended as having the right cream is vital to avoid potential harm. This is one of those times where you really must ask.

Using lube with barriers

Lubricants need to be put on after the safer sex barrier is in place. If lube is put on the body part or toy before the barrier, you're creating a slippery surface under the barrier and there is a much greater risk (almost a guarantee) of it coming/sliding off during play.

- If you're using a condom for a penis or toy to be inserted into something, put the condom on first, then the lube on the condom covered penis/toy.
- If you're using an internal condom for a vagina or anus, put the condom inside the person first, then the lube. Also, with internal condoms, the lube can also go on the thing that will penetrate, such as a toy, finger or penis before insertion.

- If you're using a condom for an individual finger, pop the condom over the finger, then put lube over the condom-covered finger.

- Regardless of treatment, if you're going to insert anything, anywhere, put a condom on it and then lube on the condom. This is an extra way to ensure cleanliness and hygiene and also makes cleaning the toy/object/person much easier.

Gloves

Gloves are a wonderful and versatile safer sex item. If you're playing with someone's genitals/anus and feel you have dirt under your fingernails or perhaps some cuts and abrasions on your hand/fingers, pop some gloves on. Most importantly, is to mention that gloves don't remove all sensory feedback, as the person wearing gloves, you can still feel plenty.

Gloves also feel excellent on skin, for the person being touched. They're just another way to explore and enjoy new and different sensory experiences. There are several types of gloves, vinyl, latex or Nitrile. Nitrile gloves are easily accessed online and are great for people who have a latex allergy.

10. LOSS OF SPONTANEITY

I honestly could not count the number of people I've heard mention that they wish they could go back to "the way it was", how they "want the spontaneity back".

Sure, while you're fighting cancer, you're not suddenly ripping each other's clothes off in the television commercial break. But it's not just cancer that can change our intimate patterns. This is also normal for people in longer term relationships and anyone experiencing any stressful life-event. Also, let's think about when you were having spontaneous sex, what was happening in your life? Was there more time with each other? More foreplay? More flirting? More affection? More intimacy? Less stress?

Spontaneous sex is not the only type of sex. Removing spontaneity gives way for intention. Sure, a little more planning might not get your juices flowing in an instant, but it shows love, thoughtfulness and caring. That's pretty hot! You can make planned sex and intimacy special, like an upcoming and exciting date. It gives you time to prepare, to make sure you're well rested and not hurried or rushed. This allows you to get in the right headspace, which will guarantee you a better time. Plus, planning can be a lot of fun and is totally psychological foreplay.

A sexuality educator I was listening to recently, discussing this topic brought up this question and it was another one of those 'ahaaa' moments with me. They asked "how many romantic movies show the caring, intentional long-term portions of relationships where couples spend their day 'doing life'. A film where they cook, do the dishes and crash in bed late at night exhausted after a full day's work?" I'm going to say, hardly any.

Romantic films usually show the first stages, meeting, dating, flirting, the new relationship energy, the excitement and adrenaline, and when you have time for so much fun. Life isn't always like that, but that doesn't mean you can't connect and have pleasure.

Sex can still be fun, pleasurable and connective, even if it needs a bit of planning.

11.   TIPS FOR LOVED ONES

Seeing a loved one go through cancer is tough, and so can knowing what to say or how to act. Whether you're a carer, friend, family member or partner, there are ways to offer connection without overstepping a line. And don't worry, we won't break!

I once saw a young person ask on a cancer support forum "how long after chemo until I can kiss my mother on the cheek?" This post shocked me and showed me how some of us could see someone having chemo as being 'poisonous', as being 'toxic' or 'harmful'. Yes, caution is (very) necessary and the medical team must tell you about all of the risks involved in all treatments. People undergoing chemo, surgeries, radiotherapy, we can be seen as easily hurt, fragile or dangerous, and rightly so. There are many side-effects of treatments, some of them are mental and some of them are physical. However, let's remember this: connection is always important, and even if someone's body and mind are changing, there are still ways to be there with someone.

It can understandably be hard to know what to do. It's also normal, when seeing a loved one be so unwell, to want to avoid causing any other harm and through that, create physical distance. That might look like reducing touch and physical contact, or even like possible avoidance. If you're a partner, lover, friend or carer of someone during treatment, I implore you, I beg you, to offer them touch. Treatment is damaging and also detaching. We need the treatment, yes, but we also need care, to feel connected to ourselves and to those around us. Don't be afraid of us, be cautious and curious with us. Think of it as getting into 'ask first' mode.

For simple touch, a peck on the lips or cheek? It's okay! We are not radioactive, we won't give you cancer and we won't break, if we all just take a little care. How do we know what to do or what not to do? We ask.

How to say it out loud.

- "Would you like me to take your hand?"
- "Is there any way you might like some loving/comforting touch right now?"
- "Would you like a hug?"
- "I'd love a cuddle; how does that sound to you?"
- "I'd love to connect with you, are there any sore spots I should avoid if I went in for a cuddle?"

- "I'd love to connect with you right now, is there a form of touch you would like?" (Arm around the shoulder, hand holding, hug from behind, foot massage and more.)
- "I love you and want to offer you affection, is there anything that would comfort you at the moment?"
- "I miss you, but I'm worried I'll hurt you if I squeeze you too hard. Is there a way I can snuggle into you?"
- "I'm wanting to show you love and affection, such as a kiss on the lips or cheek, how do you feel about that?"
- "I'm checking you out right now, fancy a kiss?"

If you're being made an offer of connection and it's not a good time? I offer some examples shortly on ways to navigate that, however a simple, "thank you, but I'm not quite up for it at the moment" is perfect. Even if the person receiving this offer is not up for it right then, you're showing love, care, concern for their well-being and the desire to remain connected. It means the world.

Not in the mood?

Whether you're the person with cancer or the partner of, there will be times when you don't feel like being intimate with others, that is fine, that is normal, that is understandable. There will also be times when you feel like connecting somehow, but aren't sure how. There are lots of places to start: Get in the bath and relax or wrap yourself in blankets with a hot-water bottle, maybe touch your body, snuggle a pet with your favourite film, ask the person you're with to intertwine your legs while you both sit on the couch or lean into their chest. During treatments, you're not going to want intimacy or touch all of the time, so feel free to let loved ones know how you're feeling and speak up in the moments it seems plausible. If you do receive an offer of intimacy and connection and you're not up for it? Remember, that's okay, that's fine, that's normal. But also remember to say thanks for the offer and be kind when you say no thanks, because you want the offers to keep coming!

How to say it out loud.

- "Thank you, that sounds amazing, it's not the best moment, can we see how I'm going later?" (Or tomorrow, or after lunch)

- "Thanks, I'm feeling quite nauseous/tired/some pain, for the moment I need to sit still, can we maybe connect later or another day?"

- "I'm really not feeling well, I'd like to sit alone for a while. Thank you so much for offering a cuddle, rain-check?"

- "I'd love to kiss you, but my mouth is a bit sore at the moment, would you like some soft neck touch instead?"

- "I'd love a hug, thank you, could you be careful around my arm? It's a bit sore."

- "I don't think I'm up for a hug right now, would you like to hold my hand?"

- "I'm pretty low on energy at the moment, but something soft and gentle would be lovely, like a snuggle?"

- Or if you're ADHD and ridiculously blunt like me "Thanks for the offer of a kiss, I'm currently trying not to vomit in my mouth, so will need to rain-check" (we both had a giggle at that).

To those undergoing treatments, if you feel your partner/lover/friend is avoiding you, unattracted to you and doesn't want to touch you? They may just be thinking they are protecting you, avoiding potentially hurting you or feel like they're pestering/pressuring you, so are pulling away. Be the one to communicate and offer a connection. Offer to snuggle, offer to touch their back while they're standing next to you, ask for a long hug hello, it guides them, and can lead to further connections. It meant the world to me, having my hand held and legs entwined on the couch with a cup of tea and chats. It was meaningful and intimate, that at times was my sex. Simple things like that were so important, and I know is/was to others during treatments.

12. FOR MY FELLOW RAINBOW-FLAGGERS

For people in the LGBTQIA+ community, medical institutions can be very difficult. I remember sitting in the chemo-chair with my then partner holding my hand. The nurse approached and looked at us holding hands, then looking at her said "oh, isn't that sweet you're such good *friends*". I know the nurse meant well, but it was devaluing to me and my partner. I did not feel like I was seen as a person, nor my partner respected. I also did not have the energy to continually educate everyone around me all day every day and advocate for who I am and for others. It's exhausting and with cancer, I didn't have it in me. So, I withdrew and I became reluctant to share my personal story with most clinicians. This is particularly important for people with cancers such as prostate, testicular, cervix, ovaries or breast (just to name a few), as these cancers are *very* gendered. Due to this people can isolate themselves from the supports that are out there as they may feel unwelcome or unseen. Speaking personally, the 'sisterhood' is very strong in breast cancer and as a non-binary person, was difficult to ignore. I avoided so many (pretty much all) support networks due to this as I did not feel welcome. If you're someone who resonates with this, if you belong to communities that are marginalised, I ask you to reach out. Reach out to that one person on your treating team you can have an honest, non-shaming conversation with. Reach out to the nurse asking for any resources the hospital knows of that are accessible and inclusive. Reach out to a friend, to find a cancer support group near you or online that is gender aware, recognises pronouns, alternative relationship models, and partnerships that are not only heterosexual. They are out there, but you may need help finding them. Feeling safe and supported is everything.

RESOURCES

Because there's limited work on sexuality and cancer and well, actual realistic and accessible sexuality education in general, resources can be hard to find. So, here are some, of varied mediums depending on what suits you best.

The 'A Better Normal' mini-book series

Available globally on Amazon in paperback or eBook format, you can search by author 'Tess Devèze' or by book title.

If you're needing support, practical solutions and guidance on more specific side-effects, or looking for help regarding a specific treatment, the 'A Better Normal' mini-book series covers quite a range.

Books in the 'A Better Normal' mini-book series are:

- 'A Better Normal for **Libido**; Your Guide to Rediscovering Intimacy After Cancer'
- 'A Better Normal for **Vaginal Dryness & Pain**; Your Guide to Rediscovering Intimacy After Cancer'
- 'A Better Normal for **Body Confidence**; Your Guide to Rediscovering Intimacy After Cancer'

- 'A Better Normal for **Chemotherapy**; Your Guide to Rediscovering Intimacy After Cancer'
- 'A Better Normal for **Hormone Therapy**; Your Guide to Rediscovering Intimacy After Cancer'
- 'A Better Normal for **Fatigue**; Your Guide to Rediscovering Intimacy After Cancer'
- 'A Better Normal for **Changes in Erection**; Your Guide to Rediscovering Intimacy After Cancer'
- 'A Better Normal for **Radiotherapy**; Your Guide to Rediscovering Intimacy After Cancer'
- 'A Better Normal for **Pain**; Your Guide to Rediscovering Intimacy After Cancer'

The all-in-one resource, 'A Better Normal; Your Guide to Rediscovering Intimacy After Cancer'

Available globally on Amazon in paperback or eBook, you can search via author 'Tess Devèze' or by book title.

If you liked the information in this book, but feel you need guidance on more, the book 'A Better Normal; Your Guide to Rediscovering Intimacy After Cancer' has all of the information included in the entire mini-book series and more. It's your one stop shop for everything you need to know about sexuality and cancer, in the one book.

Vulva Pleasure Masterclass

(connectable.podia.com/vulva-masterclass)

For anyone with a vulva who is experiencing pain and dryness, or is experiencing loss of sensation, pleasure, arousal and orgasm. This online Masterclass teaches vulva massage, which can be done on yourself or with a partner. Through massage and neurological concepts, things like arousal and pleasure can be recovered while helping heal tissues through increasing blood-flow with massage. This Masterclass is also suitable for people with vaginismus and vulvodynia.

Penis Pleasure Masterclass

(connectable.podia.com/penis-pleasure)

For anyone with a penis who is experiencing changes in erection and orgasm, or is experiencing loss of sensation, function and pleasure. This online Masterclass teaches soft penis massage, which can be done on yourself or with a partner. Through massage and neurological concepts, things like sensation and pleasure can be recovered while helping recover erectile function through increasing blood-flow with massage. This Masterclass is particularly beneficial for people post prostatectomy.

A libido and intimacy recovery program for couples

'Connection & Cancer: Reclaim Your Intimacy & Desire'.
(connectable.podia.com/libido-after-cancer)

If you would like personal support through the exact process of *how* to recover your pleasure, intimacy and libido, then this is for you. It's with me online guiding you every step of the way, and is done in the privacy of your own home. Filled with information, fun and practical solutions that I take you through for libido recovery. The people who I've worked with in this program are having life-changing results. It's an absolute honour to guide people to recover what they felt was lost forever.

'ConnectAble Therapies' (connectabletherapies.com)

For consultations and further resources on sex, intimacy & cancer.

Facebook global support group: *'Intimacy and Cancer'.* This group is for any cancer, any gender and is a very supportive space.

Instagram '@connectable_therapies', where I regularly share helpful information.

YouTube Channel on sex, intimacy & cancer: type *"Intimacy and Cancer CHANNEL"* to find it.

If you prefer video formats over reading (as cancer-brain & reading don't go well together), this YouTube Channel is filled with short videos discussing all things sex, intimacy and cancer.

'ConnectAble Courses' (connectable.podia.com)

A site of intimacy and cancer online courses for sexual recovery. Including the Masterclasses, libido recovery program and webinar mentioned here.

Intimacy & Cancer Information Webinar

(connectable.podia.com/webinar-intimacyaftercancer)

A free information webinar discussing the impacts cancer treatments have on intimacy and sexuality. It has a particular focus on libido and how it can be recovered.

Other amazing resources:

'A Touchy Subject' (atouchysubject.com)

For people with prostate cancer or experiencing changes in erection. Victoria Cullen is *the* person to go to, about sexuality and intimacy post a prostate cancer diagnosis. She also has a YouTube channel and through her website access to free resources and rehabilitation programs.

'The Art of The Hook Up' (artofthehookup.com)
This site from dating expert and communication extraordinaire is by Georgie Wolf. Not cancer specific, but incredibly on-point and with relative information for anyone struggling with the dating scene. She has podcasts, blogs, eBooks and more. She's also a workshop facilitator and a bit of a superstar here in Australia!

'Curious Creatures' (curiouscreatures.biz)
For online workshops and much more education on self-development and sexuality. They provide articles, podcasts and streamable workshops which are all very practical and very accessible. I have the privilege to work for this company, their work is changing lives.

'Bump'n Joystick' (getbumpn.com)
An intimacy aid designed for people with impaired upper limb and fine-motor function. Suitable for all genders and is flexible to varied body shapes. This toy was designed by the global disability and OT community, and it's pretty

incredible.

'The Ziggy' (luddi.co)

Another intimacy aid designed for people with limited upper limb and intact fine-motor function. Designed by the disability community and healthcare professionals, this is a multi-purpose vibrator for all genders. It's also able to be used while in a wheelchair, so is a wonderfully accessible item.

Pelvic and sexual health osteopath

For those who live in Melbourne, Australia, we have one of the top pelvic health osteopaths you'll ever find. Dr Andrew Carr from the *'Whole Being Health Collective'* is referred to as *'the body whisperer'* in clinical and sexual health circles. He works with the entire body, however has expertise and clinical focus on pelvic and sexual health. In particular, people experiencing pelvic pain including after treatments, vaginismus, atrophy and is trauma informed.

If you're not located in Melbourne, there are pelvic floor osteopaths, physiotherapists and OTs all over the world. Simply search online "Pelvic floor osteopath/physio/OT (insert the name of your city/town here)". You'll find someone near you.

Support groups in your area

If you search in google "Cancer Support (insert city/town where you live here)", there should be a list of businesses and companies that have programs near you. Some online or in person. They mightn't be sexuality specific, but there is always opportunity for discussions and learning.

ACKNOWLEDGEMENTS

For anyone and everyone out there affected by cancer, this book is for you. There can be so much to consider, to have to endure, to have to keep track of, that many parts of life take a back seat. Thank you for caring about your intimacy and connections during such a time, be it connections with yourself or with others. I hope you're supported and I truly hope there is something in this book for you.

I'm forever grateful to my clients and the thousands I support online who so openly and vulnerably share their struggles, and also their triumphs with me. This book would not exist without you. I'm inspired and amazed by you all, daily.

Thank you, to my partners and carers over the years Rog, Robi and Kane, my family and my global network of friends. There were some very dark places during treatments and you all got me through. To my booby buddies (my breast care nurses) Claire & Monique, you're my angels. Ricky Dick my oncologist - you're simply the best (Tina Turner style!) and to my RADelaidies.

Lastly, to acknowledge the incredible ethics, values and approaches to sexuality and communication from

Roger Butler at Curious Creatures (and their generosity with sharing their content with me), the occupational therapy & sexuality community (yeah OT-siggers!) and the revolutionary perspectives and therapeutic trainings I received from Deej & Uma, at the Institute of Somatic Sexology (ISS).

ABOUT THE AUTHOR

Tess Devèze is an occupational therapist (OT) having completed their bachelor degree in Melbourne Australia, founding ConnectAble Therapies, a community sexuality OT and sexology clinic focussing on sexuality and intimacy for people with neurological conditions, cancer, chronic illness and disability. They have also completed certification and trainings via the Institute of Somatic Sexology. Alongside being a sexuality OT, Tess is also a sexuality educator & workshop facilitator, and has facilitated and educated thousands of people in the topics of communication, consent, sexuality, pleasure and relationship dynamics for nearing a decade. Tess founded the global online initiative 'Intimacy and Cancer', an online support space for people of all cancers and genders to access sexual support.

As a non-binary, queer, disabled person living with cancer, Tess's work is inclusive and advocates for sexual rights for disabled, neurodivergent, gender queer/diverse and LGBTQIA+, communities, which they proudly belong to.

Tess was diagnosed with stage 3 breast cancer at the age of 36 and is still undergoing treatments.

Find them at www.connectabletherapies.com

DID YOU ENJOY THE BOOK?

As an independent author, my work survives through your support. There are so many people affected by cancer, suffering in silence. With each review or word-of-mouth recommendation you make, we can reach the many out there who are struggling and need support.

Please leave a review by visiting where you purchased this book. It's just 1 minute of your time, but could be the thing that helps this reach someone who needs it, someone who needs a better normal too.

Got feedback? Please leave a review! Plus, I'd love to hear from you. You can reach me via email at tess@connectabletherapies.com or via Instagram @connectable_therapies.